Medical Education in Early
New York

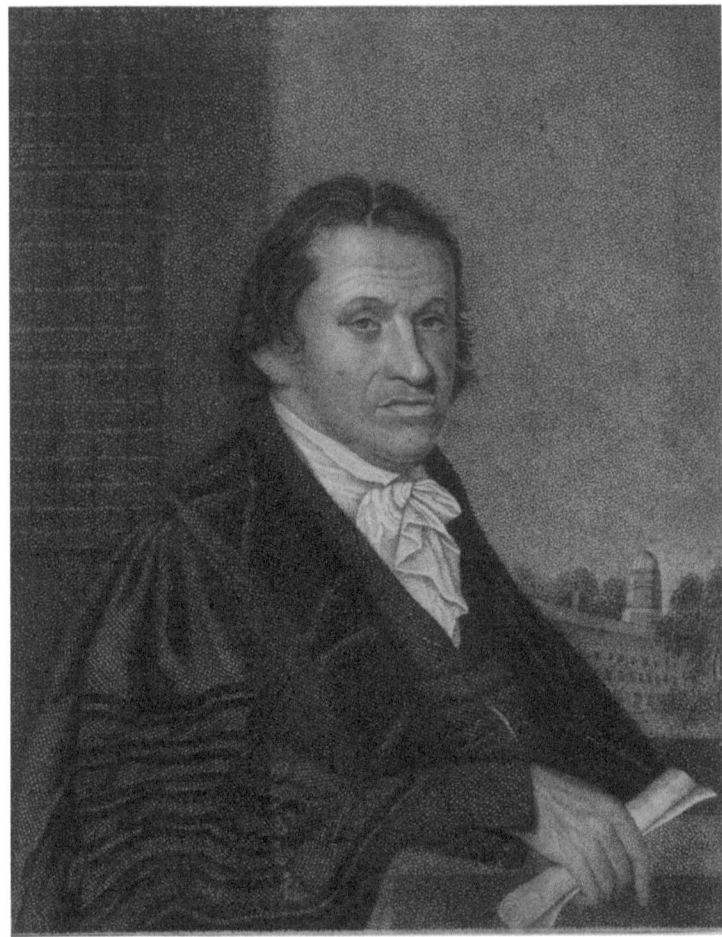

SAMUEL BARD, M.D., LL.D.

From "A Domestic Narrative of the Life of Samuel Bard, M.D., LL.D., late President of the College of Physicians and Surgeons of the University of the State of New York, &c." By Rev. John M'Vickar, A.M., Professor of Moral Philosophy and Rhetoric, Columbia College, New York. New York: Published at the Literary Rooms, corner of Broadway and Pine-Street. A Paul, Printer. 1822. King's College in the background.

Two Discourses

Dealing with

Medical Education in Early New York

By

SAMUEL BARD, M.D.

Professor of the Practice of Medicine in King's College
Later President of the College of Physicians
and Surgeons

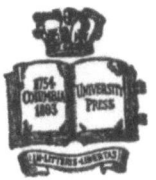

New York
COLUMBIA UNIVERSITY PRESS
1921

INTRODUCTION

At a time when Columbia University is undertaking a long step forward in the better organization of medical education and research, and when the Society of the New York Hospital is celebrating the one hundred and fiftieth anniversary of its organization, it is appropriate that there should be reprinted for the information of this generation the prophetic "Discourse upon the Duties of a Physician; with some Sentiments upon the Usefulness and the Necessity of a Public Hospital," delivered before the President and Governors of King's College at the commencement held on May 16, 1769, by Dr. Samuel Bard, Professor of the Practice of Medicine in King's College, and also the discourse on medical education delivered at the medical commencement of the College of Physicians and Surgeons on April 6, 1819 when Dr. Bard was President of that College.

The story of Dr. Samuel Bard's life is told in an address by Dr. Henry William Ducachet delivered before the New York Historical Society, August 14, 1821, and reprinted at Philadelphia in October, 1821 from the fourth volume of the American Medical Recorder. Of Huguenot descent, Dr. Bard was born in Philadelphia on April 1, 1742 and in due time became the chief practitioner of medicine in the City and Province of New York.

The first of the two discourses now reprinted, was delivered in 1769 "as advice to those gentlemen who then received the first medical degrees" conferred by what is now Columbia University. These two addresses, and particularly the first address, speak for themselves. They establish Dr. Bard's leadership in medical education in America and justify his reputation as prophet and seer.

Dr. Bard lived to be seventy-nine years of age and died on May 25, 1821. Of the early years of King's College and Columbia College Dr. Bard was a chief ornament. He served not only as Professor of the Theory and Practice of Medicine, but later as Professor of Chemistry as well as of Natural Philosophy and Astronomy. From 1787 to 1804 he was a Trustee of the College.

NICHOLAS MURRAY BUTLER

March 1, 1921

I

A DISCOURSE UPON THE DUTIES OF A PHYSICIAN

Delivered before the President and Governors of King's College at the Commencement held on the 16th day of May, 1769.

II

A DISCOURSE ON MEDICAL EDUCATION

Delivered at the Medical Commencement of the College of Physicians and Surgeons on the 6th of April, 1819.

A DISCOURSE
UPON THE
DUTIES OF A PHYSICIAN,
WITH SOME SENTIMENTS,
ON THE
USEFULNESS AND NECESSITY
OF A
PUBLIC HOSPITAL:
DELIVERED BEFORE THE
PRESIDENT AND GOVERNORS
OF
KING's COLLEGE,
AT THE COMMENCEMENT,
Held on the 16th of MAY, 1769.

As Advice to those GENTLEMEN who then received the First MEDICAL DEGREES conferred by that UNIVERSITY.

By SAMUEL BARD, M.D.
Professor of the Practice of Medicine in KING's COLLEGE.

NEW-YORK:
Printed by A. & J. ROBERTSON, at the Corner of
BEAVER-STREET, M,DCC,LXIX.

To His EXCELLENCY
SIR HENRY MOORE, Bart.
Captain General, and Governor in Chief, in and over the *Province* of NEW-YORK, and the Territories depending thereon, in *AMERICA*, Chancellor, and Vice-Admiral of the same.

SIR,

THE favourable Sentiments you were pleased to express of the following Discourse, when it was delivered, and the very generous Warmth with which your Excellency entered into the Proposal it contains, of founding a Public Infirmary in this City, have emboldened the Author to submit it to the Consideration of the Public; and to insure it a favourable Reception, he has ventured to prefix to it your Excellency's Name; not doubting but that the same Benevolence which prompted you so generously to undertake the Cause of the Poor and
Un-

ii DEDICATION.

Unhappy, will now plead his Excuse, for the Liberty he has taken of proposing your Excellency's humane and benevolent Example, to the Imitation of his Fellow Citizens and Country Men.

May your Excellency, and every generous Contributor to this Institution, enjoy the Happiness of seeing the good Effects of your charitable Endeavours; and as the just Reward of your Humanity, may "*the Blessing of him that is ready to perish come upon you.*"

>In which Hope,
>I have the Honor to be,
>With the greatest Respect.
>Your Excellency's
>Most obedient
>Humble Servant,
>
>SAMUEL BARD.

THE PREFACE.

THE Scheme of a Public Hospital for the Reception of the poor Sick of this Government and City, is a Subject, which for a long Time paft, has employed the Attention of many charitable and benevolent Inhabitants; particularly of thofe Gentlemen engaged in the practice of Phyfic, and Offices of Religion, whofe Profeffions afford them the moft frequent Opportunities of knowing the great Neceffity there is for fuch an Inftitution.

In particular, a Plan has often been propofed, and the moft proper Method for putting it in Execution confidered, by a Set of Medical Gentlemen, who have formed themfelves into a Society for promoting the Knowledge, and extending the Ufefulnefs of their Profeffion: and it has been a Refolution entered upon the Minutes of that Society, from its firft Inftitution, that they fhould Addrefs the Legiflature upon that Subject, on the firft favourable Opportunity.

PREFACE.

It likewise has repeatedly been mentioned by the different Professors of Medicine, (particularly Doctors Middleton, and Jones,) in their public Lectures, and earnestly recommended to the Consideration of the Inhabitants; the unhappy Disputes however, in which we have lately been engaged with our Mother Country, have hitherto rendered their Endeavours fruitless; but, they nevertheless (convinced of the great Necessity there was for such an Institution, and the very great Advantages which all Orders of People must derive from it) resolved to persist in their Endeavours, until some happy Occasion should offer of pushing it with some Probability of Success. Such an Occasion now presents itself, and the Warmth and Zeal, which his Excellency the Governor, and most of his honorable Council, have expressed for it, and the Liberality, with which they have subscribed towards it, induce them to think the present, the fittest Time, for recommending it, to the serious Consideration of the Public.

And

PREFACE.

And as an Institution of this Nature, must necessarily be calculated for the Benefit of the distressed of all Sects and Persuasions whatsoever, it is hoped, that the generous and public spirited of every Denomination, will enter warmly into the Design, and promote it with that Zeal, which should actuate the Breast of every Man, who thinks it his Duty to relieve the Necessities of his Fellow Creatures, or promote the Happiness of Society

A DISCOURSE UPON THE DUTIES OF A PHYSICIAN

Homines ad Deos, nulla re proprius accedunt, quam Salutem Hominibus dando.   CICERO.

There is nothing by which a Man approaches nearer to the Perfections of the Deity, than by restoring the Sick, to the Enjoyment of the Blessings of Health.

THAT this Country has, ever since its Discovery and Settlement, laboured under the greatest Disadvantages, from the imperfect Manner, in which Students have been instructed in the Principles of Medicine; and from the Consequent prevailing Ignorance of but too many of its Professors; is a Truth which cannot be contested; and of which many unhappy Families have severely felt the fatal Effects.

The present Occasion therefore must give the most real Pleasure to every considerate Man, or Lover of his Country; and surely there is no Friend of Learning, but must rejoice to see these Gentlemen, who have given the most public and ample Testimony of their Abilities, now soliciting the Honors of this University, in a Profession hitherto (at least in a regular Manner) uncultivated amongst us.

I am therefore particularly happy in having this Opportunity of congratulating every public spirited Friend and Patron of this College, and especially those of the medical Institution, upon the present Instance of its Success, which affords so pleasing a Prospect of its rising Reputation and future Utility.

But it is to you, Gentlemen, who are Candidates for medical Degrees, that I mean in a more particular Manner to address my present Discourse; receive then my Thanks for the Honors you have already reflected upon us, and as both for your Sakes and our own, I cannot but be anxious for your future Reputation;

tation; let me once more, before we part, request your Attention for a few Moments, whilst I endeavour to explain to you the weighty duties of your Profession----A Profession, in the Practice of which, Integrity and Abilities, will place you among the most useful; and Ignorance and Dishonesty, among the most pernicious Members of Society.

And be not alarmed, if I set out with telling you, that your Labours must have no End. No less than Life, and its greatest Blessing Health, are to be the Objects of your Attention; and would you acquit yourselves to your own Consciences, you must spend *your* Days in assiduous Enquiries, after the Means of rendering those of others long and happy.

Do not therefore imagine, that from this Time your Studies are to cease; so far from it, you are to be considered as but just entering upon them; and unless your whole Lives, are one continued Series of Application and Improvement, you will fall short of your Duty. For, if in the Eye of the Law, the Man who does not afford, to all immediately under his

Care

Care and Protection, as far as in him lies, the necessary Means of preserving Life, is considered as accessary to Murder, how will that Physician excuse himself to his own Conscience, or what Palliation of his Guilt, will he plead at the awful Bar of eternal Justice, who instead of embracing and industriously cultivating every Opportunity of Improvement, shall (conscious of his own Inability) rashly tamper with the Lives of his Fellow Creatures; and, at the risk of their Safety, defraud them of their Property? Would not any one consider the Lawyer an Impostor, not to use a harsher Phrase, who, conscious of his own Ignorance, should give Advice, which might endanger the Estate of another? And is not the Physician who imposes Ignorance upon me for Knowledge, and puts my Life to the hazard of an uncertain die; so much the greater Impostor, in as much as my Life, is of greater Estimation than my Estate. In a Profession then, like that you have embraced, where the Object is of so great Importance as the Life of a Man; you are accountable even for the Errors of Ignorance, unless you have embraced every Opportunity of obtaining Knowledge.

And

And to a Man, who has any Conscience at all, it will be but a slight Alleviation of his Remorse, to say, after some fatal Blunder, *I knew no better!* Unless he can likewise add, that it is to be attributed to the Frailty of his Nature, and not to the Negligence of his Disposition, that he was not better informed. Nor will a weeping Parent receive much Consolation from this Reflection, that by the fatal Ignorance of his Physician, and not by the malignancy of the Disease, he has been robbed of the Staff and Support of his Life, the Joy and Comfort of his declining Age.

Did I know a Wretch among the Practitioners of Medicine, whose insensible Soul neither feels for the Distresses he may Occasion, nor partakes in the Joys he may give rise to; I say, did I know a Man so void of every Sentiment of Tenderness, and Humanity; I would advise him, from Motives of Interest and Gain, to endeavour at the Attainment of Skill in his Profession. But to you, Gentlemen, I will point out the Gratification inseparable from the Acquisition of Knowledge, that ever to be

wished

wished for Praise, which falls from the Lips of the Wife and the Virtuous, the Applause of an approving Conscience, and the unspeakable Pleasure of doing good, as the Reward of all your Toil, and as the strongest Spur to your future Industry.

As to those who have neither Emulation nor Honesty, who neither have Abilities, nor will give themselves the Trouble of acquiring them; I would recommend it to such, seriously to consider the Sixth Commandment,

'THOU SHALT DO NO MURDER.'

In the Prosecution of your Studies, let such Authors as have transmitted to us Observations founded upon Nature, claim your particular Attention. Of these, HIPPOCRATES shines the foremost; his unwearied Diligence in observing and collecting the Symptoms of Diseases, his Fidelity and Accuracy in relating them, his happy Facility in discovering their Causes, his almost prophetic Knowledge of their Events, and his successful Treatment of them, can never be sufficiently admired, and will hand down his Name, with Honor and Applause to the latest Posterity. A few

A few others among the Ancients, who have followed the Steps of Hippocrates, are well worth your Perusal; but whilst you acknowledge *their* Merit, do not affect the Pedantry of despising the Moderns; and carefully avoid that Rock, upon which most of the fond Admirers of Antiquity have split, a blind and slavish Attachment to its Opinions; the Bar where Truth has been so often Shipwrecked, and which more than the want of Ingenuity or Capacity, stopped the Progress of Learning for above twelve hundred Years.

Why should we give more to those Times, than they attributed to themselves? Read the Writings of the wisest among the Ancients, and they are filled with Modesty and Diffidence, why then should we ascribe to them, Infallibility and Omniscience? They doubted the Assertions, and controverted the Opinions of the Times which preceded them; why should not we doubt and controvert theirs; and leave to Posterity the Liberty of controverting ours? Let us then examine their Writings with Candour, but with Freedom, and embrace or

reject

reject their Opinions; as they shall be found consistent, or inconsistent with later Experience.

Without therefore depreciating the Merit of the Ancients, let us do Justice to their Posterity, and do not from an over Zeal for Antiquity, sacrifice Sydenham and Boerhaave, to the Manes of Hippocrates and Galen.---I see no Reason why Time only should lessen our Abilities, and surely Experience must increase our Knowledge: and although I think some of the Ancients may be read with great Advantage; yet it is the most celebrated Moderns (who with equal Abilities enjoy the additional Advantage of near 2000 Years of Experience) whom I would recommend to your most attentive Perusal; particularly those great Ornaments of their Profession, SYDENHAM, BOERHAAVE, HUXHAM, PRINGLE, and WHYTT; and some others of our latest English and Scotch Physicians, "*Horum Scripta nocturna versate manu, versate diurna.*"

In your Intercourse with your Fellow Practitioners, let Integrity, Candour, and Delicacy be be your Guides. There is a particular Sensibility of Disposition, which seems essential to delicate Honor, and which I believe is the best Counterpoise to Self-Interest. This I would by all Means advise you to cultivate, as you will meet with many Occasions where it only can direct your Conduct.

Never affect to despise a Man for the want of a regular Education, and treat even harmless Ignorance, with Delicacy and Compassion, but when you meet with it joined with foolhardiness and Presumption, you must give it no quarter.

On no Pretence whatever, practice those little Arts of Cunning and Dissimulation, which to the Scandal of the Profession, have been but too frequent amongst us. Nor ever attempt to raise your Fame on the Ruins of another's Reputation; and remember that you ought not only to be cautious of your Words, a Shrug or a Whisper, the stare of Surprise, or a piteous Exclamation of Sorrow, more effectually wound another's Reputation, and more clearly betray the Baseness of a Man's own Heart, than the loudest Expressions.

Do not pretend to Secrets, Panacea's, and Nostrums, they are illiberal, dishonest, and inconsistent with your Characters, as Gentlemen and Physicians, and with your Duty as Men--- For if you are possessed of any valuable Remedy, it is undoubtedly your Duty to divulge it, that as many as possible may reap the Benefit of it; and if not, (which is generally the Case) you are propagating a Falsehood, and imposing upon Mankind.

In your Behaviour to the Sick, remember always that your Patient is the Object of the tenderest Affection, to some one, or perhaps to many about him; it is therefore your Duty, not only to endeavour to preserve his Life, but to avoid wounding the Sensibility of a tender Parent, a distressed Wife, or an affectionate Child. Let your Carriage be humane and attentive, be interested in his Welfare, and shew your Apprehension of his Danger, rather by your Assiduity to relieve, than by any harsh or brutal Expressions of it. On the other hand, never buoy up a dying Man with groundless Expectations of Recovery, this is at best a good natured and humane Deception, but too often it arises from the baser Motives of Lucre and Avarice: besides, it is really cruel, as the stroke of Death is always most severely felt, when unexpected; and the grim Tyrant may in general be disarmed of his Terrors, and rendered familiar to the most timid, and apprehensive; either by frequent Meditation, by the Arguments of Philosophy, or by the Hopes and Promises of Religion. But even overlooking the important Concerns of Futurity; the Business of this Life may render such a Conduct highly dangerous and criminal; as those to whom the thoughts of Death are painful, are too apt when flattered with the Prospect of Recovery, to neglect the necessary Provision against a Disappointment, and by that Means involve their Families in Confusion and Distress.

Above all Things, avoid any ridiculous Expressions of Humour, at the bed-side of a sick Man; you cannot chuse a more unseasonable Opportunity for your Mirth; nor will you find a Person of a generous and benevolent Disposition, who can smile even at the Repetition of a Witticism,

Witticism, which carries with it the Appearance of so much Inhumanity.

Let your Prescriptions be simple, and as neat and agreeable as the Nature of the Remedy will permit---Nothing can be more abfurd than the Farrago of some, nothing more difguftful than the Slovenlinefs of others; for it is impoffible to learn the true Virtues of Medicines, from compound Prefcriptions; and Inelegance frequently difappoints us of their Effects.---And as it is probable, from the Mode of Practice in this Country, that you will not only be the Prefcribers, but likewife the Difpenfers of your Medicines, let your Integrity be proof againft the Temptation of unneceffarily multiplying Prefcriptions, and truft rather to the Liberality of your Patient, than to the Quantity of your Phyfic, for your Reward. For altho' perhaps by this Method you may fometimes think your Services undervalued, yet you will always enjoy the fuperior Satisfaction of confcious Rectitude, which, by an honeft Man, will ever be preferred to a trifling Emolument.---

In

In the Infancy of this Country, the present Mode of practising Medicine was necessarily introduced, from the Scarcity, both of Inhabitants and Physicians. But in so populous a City as this, it is beyond a Doubt, that the Regulations it is now under, are both injurious to the Inhabitants, and dishonorable to the Profession: yet I confess it is not very easy to point out a Remedy to the Inconveniences attendant on it. There is but one, and that perhaps at present would not be thought expedient; but until it is, those who are in good Circumstances must rely wholly upon the Integrity of their Physicians; and for the Poor who are the greatest sufferers, we must endeavour to find out some other Source of Relief.

Whenever you shall be so unhappy as to fail, in your Endeavours to relieve; let it be your constant Aim to convert, particular Misfortunes into general Blessings, by carefully inspecting the Bodies of the Dead, inquiring into the Causes of their Diseases, and thence
im-

improving your own Knowledge, and making further and useful Discoveries in the healing Art.

Nor can I help regretting the many Obstacles you will meet with in prosecuting this so necessary an Enquiry; from the Prejudices of the People in general, and a false Tenderness and mistaken Delicacy in Relations. Time and Perseverance however must overcome popular Prejudices, and will I hope before long, remove these Difficulties, and open this Door to Medical Improvement.

Let those who are at once the unhappy Victims, both of Poverty and Disease, claim your particular Attention; I cannot represent to myself a more real Object of Charity, than a poor Man with perhaps a helpless Family, labouring under the complicated Miseries of Sickness and Penury. Paint to yourselves the agonizing feelings of a Parent, whilst labouring under some painful Disease, he beholds a helpless Offspring around his Bed, in want of the necessaries of Nature; imagine the Despair of an affectionate Wife, and a tender Mother.

Mother, who can neither relieve the Pain and Anxiety of her Husband, nor supply the importunate cravings of her Children; and *then* deny them your Assistance if you can---but the Supposition is injurious to Humanity, and *you* in particular, I know want no such Incitements to Duty and Benevolence. I cannot however help regretting, the very frequent Opportunities you will meet with, particularly in this Place, of exercising your Humanity upon such Occasions; owing to the want of a proper Asylum, for such unhappy and real Objects of Charity, it is truly a reproach, that a City like this, should want a public Hospital, one of the most useful and necessary charitable Institutions that can possibly be imagined.

The labouring Poor are allowed to be the support of the Community; their Industry enables the Rich to live in Ease and Affluence, and it is from the Hands of the Manufacturer we derive, not only the Necessaries, but the Superfluities of Life; whilst the poor Pittance he earns will barely supply the Necessities of Nature, and it is literally by the sweat of his Brow, that he gains his daily Subsistance; how heavy

heavy a Calamity muſt Sickneſs be to ſuch a Man, which putting it out of his Power to work, immediately deprives him and perhaps a helpleſs Family of Bread!

Nor would the good Effects of an Hoſpital be wholly confined to the Poor, they would extend to every Rank, and greatly contribute to the Safety and Welfare of the whole Community. Every Country has its particular Diſeaſes; the Varieties of Climate, Expoſure, Soil, Situation, Trades, Arts, Manufactures, and even the Character of a People, all pave the Way to new Complaints, and vary the Appearance of thoſe, with which we are already acquainted; Hence Ægypt is ſubject to the Plague; Holland to Intermittents; the Weſt-Indies to Putrid; and the Northern Countries to inflammatory Diſeaſes; and Spain and England to Hypochondriocal Complaints; which reigning Diſeaſes of a Country, not only have Peculiarities of their own, but often vary the Characters of ſuch as are common to that Country with others, and theſe Peculiarities with their Antidotes can properly be learned only in public Hospitals, where having a number of Sick at one Time, not only affords an Opportunity of the better comparing and remarking their Symptoms, but they being under a certain Discipline and Regulation, the Faces of their diseases are not changed, either by the indulgence of friends or the officiousness of Nurses; which is too often the case in private practice. Another argument, (and that by no means the least,) for an Institution of this Nature, is, that it affords the best and only means of properly instructing Pupils in the Practice of Medicine; as far therefore, as the breeding good and able Physicians, which in all Countries and at all Times has been thought an object of the highest Importance, deserves the Consideration of the Public, this Institution must likewise claim its Protection and Encouragement.

Nor is the Scheme of a Public Hospital I believe so impracticable, nor the Execution of it, I hope at so great a distance, as at first sight it may appear to be. There are Numbers in this Place I am sure (was a Subscription once set on foot,
upon

upon an extensive and generous Plan) whose Fortunes enable them, and whose Benevolence would prompt them, liberally to contribute to so useful an Institution; it wants but a Prime Mover, whose Authority would give Weight to the Undertaking, and whose Zeal and Industry, would promote it. Such a one I hope e'er long to see rise up amongst us, and may the Blessing of the Poor, and the Applause of the Good and Humane, be the Reward of his Assiduity and Labour.

F I N I S.

DISCOURSE

ON

MEDICAL EDUCATION

DELIVERED AT THE

MEDICAL COMMENCEMENT

OF

THE COLLEGE OF PHYSICIANS AND SURGEONS

OF THE

UNIVERSITY OF THE STATE OF NEW-YORK,

ON THE

SIXTH OF APRIL, 1819.

BY SAMUEL BARD, M. D. LL. D.

President of the College.

NEW-YORK:
Printed by C. S. Van Winkle, Printer to the University,
No. 101 Greenwich Street.
....
1819.

DISCOURSE

ON

MEDICAL EDUCATION.

———•———

GENTLEMEN,

A sound mind, in a sound body, constitutes the principal happiness and perfection of man; the means, therefore, by which such great and essential benefits are to be secured, have ever been the object of his solicitude, and most anxious inquiry. Bountiful nature has placed both, to a certain degree, within our reach; but she has not offered them gratuitously to our acceptance; and if we would enjoy, we must consent to purchase them, at the price which she has invariably set upon these, and all other blessings, she pours so profusely around us. That price, (young gentlemen, I address myself particularly to you,) that price is *persevering industry, and well-directed labour*; without which, nothing great or excellent was ever attained; but when properly aided by these, it is not easy to set limits to the powers of man, or to say, what he may not atchieve. Nor is this universal law of our nature more applicable to the health of the body than it is to the improvement of the mind; every exercise of which " upon the theorems of science, (says the admirable author of Hermes,) tends to call forth and strengthen our native and original vigour. Be the subject immediately productive or not, the nerves of reason are braced by mere employ, and we become better actors in the drama of life, whether our parts be of the sedate or the active kind."

Man, in every state of society, is obliged to acknowledge this truth. It is only in the ends he has in view, in the variety of things which he deems good and useful, that the untutored savage differs from the civilized man—that the ignorant and the vicious differ from the wise and the good. The means by which the objects of their pursuit are acquired, are the same in both. " It is as easy to become a scholar, as it is to become a gamester, or any other character equally low and illiberal: the same application, the same quantity of habit, will fit us for the one, as completely as for the other."* Indeed, we are, in a peculiar degree, the creatures of habit, and it is as easy to establish good and useful, as it is to establish evil and pernicious, habits. Hence the great value and importance of education; that such talents and faculties as God and nature have given us, may not only be called forth, but restricted within proper limits. and directed to their proper objects: to private happiness, and to the public good. Otherwise, like seed committed to a fertile soil, but not enlivened by a genial sun, they may lie buried and inactive forever; or if not restrained by due culture, they will shoot out into wild and luxuriant branches, which will never produce good and wholesome fruit. For man is an active and a restless being; nothing becomes so insupportable to him as continued inaction; if he is not doing good, he will probably be engaged in evil; he will

*Harris.

do mischief rather than do nothing. Even the savage, to whom rest is the most dignified, as well as the most grateful, enjoyment, continually has recourse to the laborious toils of the chase, or to the fatiguing dangers of war, to relieve himself from the irksome feelings of protracted quiet; thus, too, in civilized life, all the envied qualities of great genius and brilliant talents are ever at work on good or evil. When unimproved by study, and unrestrained by discipline, they too frequently, like a wandering and a blazing meteor, burn and destroy every thing they approach; but when restricted in their course by proper principles, and directed by wisdom and virtue, they warm, and cherish, and illuminate, like the blessed sun. It is, therefore, in the constitution of our frame, and in the nature and structure of our minds, that we discover the reason and truth of the maxim, that the happiness of private life, the peace of society, and the stability of government, especially of all free governments, depends upon the instruction, information, and correct habits, of the people. To give these their proper direction, and to establish them firmly, we must begin with early youth; we must lay the foundation of all professional excellence, correct morals, and pure religion, as well as of good government, in our common schools. From whence, otherwise, shall offices be filled with ability; where shall we find just magistrates, and able teachers of religion and virtue; where the protectors of our rights and our property; where the preservers of our health and our lives; where, in short, good citizens, if we neglect to instruct our youth, and leave them to grope their devious way without a guide through the labyrinth of this mazy world?

But general observations on the necessity and advantage of education, cannot be very necessary before this audience; let us, therefore, turn our attention to that branch of learning, to which this College is particularly devoted, and after considering the necessary preparation, endeavour to explain the nature of such institutions and discipline as experience has proved to be useful and requisite in the education of an accomplished physician and surgeon.

It has of late been made a question, sanctioned by some great names, particularly in this country, how far the study of the Greek and Latin languages is necessary, or even useful, in either of the learned professions, excepting that of Divinity. But yielding, for the present, the argument for their absolute necessity, I believe it may be said with great truth, that there is no study or discipline, in which a boy, who is intended for any liberal profession, not excepting merchandise, which is the most general—or who may take a part in the government of his country, to which, with us, all may aspire—can, from the age of eight years to that of sixteen or eighteen, be employed, so generally and truly useful, as classical learning. The study of grammar, and the application of its rules, as practised in a good school, form, perhaps, the very best exercise that can be invented, to rouse the ambition, to quicken the apprehension, to ripen the judgment, and to establish a habit of close and diligent application, the first and the greatest lesson of life. And the youth who can read Homer and Virgil, Plato and Cicero, without imbibing some of their noble and generous sentiments, without having his judgment strengthened, his taste refined, and his heart mended, must be strangely deficient in all good feeling, or in any improvable faculty of mind. The elements, therefore, of classical learning may justly be considered, and have been proved by long experience, to be the best preparation for any employment above those of the mechanic arts; and before it is time to begin the study of either of the learned professions, or to enter a counting house, a young man may easily acquire these, together with a correct knowledge of his own language, and so much mathematical learning as is necessary and useful in the ordinary business of life. As to the modern languages, their great utility in the commerce of the world cannot be denied: but in forming the character, an object of far greater consequence, they certainly fall very far below the ancient languages; nor can any person, who will consider how much the knowledge of one language facilitates the acquisition of another, and how much more the knowledge of two facilitates that of a third, think, even in this respect, the time lost, which is spent in acquiring the Latin, the root and origin of the Italian, Spanish, and French, languages.

But farther; languages are the repositories of science; losing a language, therefore, is like the destruction of an immense library, which cannot be replaced If the originals are neglected purposely, the copies may be accidentally lost, by the ravages of a barbarous foe, or the lapse of time, and thus by neglecting a language, one means of perpetuating knowledge, so far as that language is concerned, is certainly lost. Besides, though science may be translated, taste and talent cannot. The spirit of original composition is too volatile to be transfused; to catch it, we must ascend to the fountain head.

Although, therefore, we acknowledge that every thing really necessary in the theory and practice of medicine, may be learned from the excellent authors who have written originally in English; and that all the best works of other languages are to be had correctly translated into our own, still, as it is not very becoming for a professional man to be totally ignorant of those languages in which all the ancient records of his art are preserved, and from which all the technical terms of which he is in the daily use are derived; it is hoped that classical learning will again assume its place, if not as absolutely necessary, at least as very useful, and highly ornamental, in the character of a physician.

The great error in our system of education is, that we are too much in a hurry, and that our young men are ushered into the world, and commence the practice of their professions, at a period so early, and after a preparation so slight, that very few have acquired the prudence or the knowledge requisite to govern their conduct in either; and hence arise the errors and failure of too many, and our general, and I am afraid I may say, too just, reputation for superficial attainments. Could we keep our youth at school until sixteen, at college until twenty, and in a counting house, or at the study of the professions, until twenty-four or twenty-five years of age, they would be more generally successful in life ; we should have fewer failures in trade, and more respectability and eminence in our professional men. Am I asked how it happens that in our own profession the general practice is so widely different? I can only answer, it is a state which we rather submit to than approve; that for the present we must palliate a disease we cannot immediately cure ; that such is the condition of medicine throughout this widely extended, and thinly inhabited country, that very few of its practitioners can be compensated for an expensive education; and that the interest of the people, as well as the utility of the profession, are better promoted by sending abroad a considerable number of young men, decently, but competently initiated in the principles of their art, than only a few of higher qualifications. But this state of things is rapidly changing––perhaps has hitherto been unavoidable ; and a just apology for it may be found in the infancy of our country, and its recent emancipation from a state of thraldom and dependence.

I rejoice, therefore, to see, and congratulate my

fellow-citizens on, the change. Many able advocates for the good old discipline have lately risen up among us, and a great and manifest improvement, in this respect, has already been made, and is rapidly progressing, in our schools and colleges.

A classical education is a fine preparation for acting in society with complacence, propriety, and dignity; for sound learning, and correct taste, are nearly connected with pure morals: independent of all principle, they undoubtedly give a delicacy and sensibility to the mind, very favourable to virtue ; and whilst they are, in themselves, a prominent source of happiness to the individual, and place him above the necessity of seeking it from sources less pure, they, at the same time, become the means of diffusing happiness around him. "A wise and able magistrate, a learned professor of the law, a humane and benevolent physician, no less than an enlightened teacher of religion, contribute to the happiness of posterity, as well as that of the age in which they live: by their knowledge, they mitigate the evils of their cotemporaries; by their example, they mend the characters of those with whom they associate; and, by their precepts, they sow the seeds of excellence which may bless and exalt their country to future generations."

Medicine is a comprehensive and an intricate science, founded on numberless facts which have been discovered through the successive periods of distant ages, and which have been collected and preserved in the writings of almost innumerable authors, of different nations and tongues. It has necessarily been coloured and disfigured by the credulity of some; rejected, lost, and again revived, by the cautious discrimination of others; elucidated by new discoveries, and confirmed by later experience. Among ignorant and barbarous nations, this science has ever been connected with religion, involved in mystery, and disfigured by superstition. As men advanced from barbarism, it assumed a more rational form, and, resting on the solid basis of experience, under the polished Greeks, directed by the genius of Hippocrates, acquired beauty, symmetry, and strength: until, as the refinements of a speculative philosophy began to prevail, theoretic opinions were substituted for fact and experiment; the subtlety of the schools, and the wanderings of the imagination, for sound reasoning and chaste deduction. By these errors, the progress of medical science, though not absolutely arrested, was greatly checked; until, through the important discovery of the circulation of the blood, by Harvey, and the introduction of a strict philosophy, by Bacon, in which opinion was made to give place to observation, and a patient investigation of facts was substituted for the quibbles of sophistry, the science of medicine became again placed on its proper basis—nature, observation, and experience. From this moment, anatomy, chemistry, natural history, and natural philosophy, which, although they had long been in the train of medicine, had rather followed, than directed her researches, were impressed into her service, and made to take the lead in a medical education; nor until he has made considerable progress in these, can the student of medicine be properly qualified even to begin what is the great object of his pursuit, the study of diseases, and their cure.

In a profession so various, so intricate, and so expensive, it is easy to see that the scholar can make but little progress by private study. Lost and bewildered in the multiplicity of objects, and in the contrariety of conflicting opinions, he absolutely requires the hand of a master to lead him into the plainest and most direct path; to remove, as he goes along, the obstacles which may obstruct his progress; and to point out such as are most worthy his observation. Nor are there many individuals who are qualified to teach all the preliminary branches; each of them is sufficiently extensive to employ the time, and occupy the attention, of a man of no common attainments.

Besides, chemistry requires a laboratory; botany a garden; and anatomy a theatre and subjects; and, above all, the nature of diseases, and the practice of medicine, cannot be taught but in a public hospital. Much, therefore, as oral instruction, and the voice of a professor, are to be preferred to the silent investigations of the closet, still more is required: the co-operation of several teachers, and the facilities of a public institution and thus, too, in a large city, where only, in this country at least, anatomy and the practice of medicine can be properly taught. In both these branches, the student must not only receive the instructions of his teacher—he must not only reflect on and digest what he hears and reads, but he must see, and handle, and examine, for himself. In anatomy, the subject, properly prepared, must be placed before him; without this, the most accurate description, even when aided by the finest plates and drawings, will be found wholly inadequate to convey correct ideas, or to make durable impressions on his mind. The parts must be unfolded by the knife; they must be distended by injections; and whatever is uninteresting, and obscures their intimate structure, must be removed; or the student will look with a vacant eye, upon what, to him at least, will appear an unformed mass: and if possible, after having been taught what he is to look for, and what is most worthy his observation, he should handle the knife and the syringe for himself—he should learn how to prepare the subject for the instruction of others.

In chemistry, the science of nature, by which we are admitted into her confidence, are taught her secrets, and learn her processes, but slow progress can be made without a teacher, aided, too, by a large and expensive apparatus; for although by the introduction of a more correct language, and a more liberal philosophy, all the jargon and mystery in which the old chemists clothed their communications, and concealed their art, have been done away; still, the multiplicity of facts, the delicacy of processes, and the variety of apparatus, are such, that practice only can give that dexterity which is necessary to ensure success; and to acquire this dexterity unassisted, would require more time, and be accompanied by greater expense, than most students of medicine could well afford.

In botany and natural history, the number of objects to be examined, and with which it is necessary to become acquainted, is so great, that without a garden and a museum, without arrangement and system, no correct or valuable knowledge can be acquired.

And, lastly, in the study of diseases, and in the practice of medicine, no histories, however accurate—no reasoning, however just—can convey the knowledge necessary for their treatment and cure. The student must see, and hear, and feel for himself. The hue of the complexion the feel of the skin, the lustre or languor of the eye, the throbbing of the pulse and the palpitations of the heart, the quickness and ease of respiration, and the tone and tremor of the voice, the confidence of hope, and the despondence of fear, as they are expressed in the countenance, baffle all description; and yet all and each of these convey important and necessary information. Where can these be learned but at the bedsides of the sick? and where shall a young man, who cannot be admitted into the privacies of families, or the chambers of women, acquire this necessary information, but in a public hospital, which is not only intended as an asylum to relieve the complicated misery of poverty and sickness, but as a school of medicine, to contribute to the public welfare; and, as such, deserves and receives the patronage of government, even more than as a mere charitable institution.

But beside these considerations, and the impossibility of teaching medicine in private, there are many advantages which attend public institutions in this, as well as most other sciences: one, is, that from the division of the subject, a more enlarged, comprehensive, and systematic view of the whole will be taken; its connection with, and dependence on, other branches of learning, will be more clearly pointed out; and general laws and fundamental principles will be better taught.

The student learns what are the proper objects of his inquiry at each stage, and, as he goes along, is taught how to make a proper use of his previous acquirements and experience.

Besides, young men engaged in the same studies, mutually assist each other; emulation, which warms and engages the passions on the side of whatever is excellent, cannot be excited without rivals; without emulation in the scholar, instruction will proceed but with a languid pace, and excellence is never attained. Nor is emulation confined to the scholar. The emoluments of the teacher depend on his fame, and both on his talents and industry. Stimulated, therefore, by his interest, and spurred on by his ambition, he will make every exertion to recommend his lectures which he knows are to be brought to the ordeal of a nice and critical examination. Among his hearers, there will always be a number of the elder students, very able to judge of his merits, and very willing to discover his errors. Such a system of education cannot long be conducted in a slovenly or incompetent manner; negligence will sit very uneasily in it, and incompetence cannot long keep her seat in a professor's chair.

Nor is it by exciting their emulation only, that young men, assembled in a public school, are of use to each other; they mutually instruct one another, by their daily conversation, and in societies formed for the purpose of discussing professional opinions, on which they often exercise a degree of attention and acuteness which serves as no inadequate test of their truth and usefulness; and this farther serves to explain them to their understandings, and fix them in their memories, with more clearness and precision than hearing them many times repeated from their professors.

Indolence is the greatest enemy to learning; but indolence is a vice bred and nourished in solitude, and can hardly exist at a public school, but in minds of so heavy a mould as to be incapable of culture. But dissipation is the error into which a young man of lively disposition and quick parts, especially on first coming from the retirement of the country into a large and luxuriant city, is most apt to fall; and unless he possess some strength of mind, the variety of new scenes, the novelty of surrounding objects, and the allurements of pleasure, too frequently seize upon his imagination, occupy his thoughts, waste his time and his resources, blast his own prospects, and disappoint the hopes and expectations of his friends. Against this I have nothing to urge but the common, though strong and irresistible, argument of duty and necessity; nor any remedy to propose, but that of wholesome employment. It is at the commencement of your career that you will be in the greatest danger; if you postpone your indulgence for a short time, even for a few weeks, until you are fairly engaged in your studies, full occupation will at least lessen the temptation; and when once you see how absolutely incompatible dissipation and pleasure are with duty and improvement, you will probably find yourselves able to resist their attractions, or, I should rather hope, they will have no attractions for you.

On the other hand, to continue in retirement, and there to labour without plan or design, may indeed accumulate a confused mass of materials; but beauty, order, and proportion, are the result of skill: he that would build a palace, must employ an architect. So the student of medicine, who trusts to his own unassisted researches, or who is directed by an inadequate guide, may load his memory and confound his judgment, by a great number of facts, and a medley of opinions, which will only lead him into error, and end at last in darkness and confusion. But he who is properly initiated into the rudiments of his art, pursues his improvement in the light of day; every step he takes, brings him nearer to his purposed end; every fact and opinion he learns, takes its proper place; and knowledge—clear, precise, and accurate knowledge, is the happy result.

In no profession are sound learning, clear and definite opinions, and correct conduct, of more consequence, than in that of medicine; in the exercise of which, our dearest interests, our health and lives, and the health and lives of our parents, wives, children, and friends, are deeply and essentially concerned. For let it be remembered, that there is no middle course in medicine: it is a mistake, to suppose the conduct of a physician is ever of that neutral and inconsequential nature, that although it do no good, it will do but little harm. If, through ignorance, a physician does not do good, he will probably do much injury; for our opportunities of acting are so fleeting, that they must be seized at the moment; and to lose time is, frequently, to do all we can to render the case under our care desperate or fatal. Nor, on the contrary, is there any profession, in which that cautious diffidence, which is the result of deep knowledge, is of greater consequence, than in that of the physician. In our profession, to know when to act with vigour, when to palliate symptoms, or to look on with patience, and from what circumstances to draw our indications, is the result only of a thorough knowledge of our subject; nor in any profession is that meddling presumption, which is ever the companion, and most frequently the veil of ignorance, more dangerous.

Nor are the happy consequences of a good education, in medicine, confined to the chambers of the sick; a physician must always, in some measure, become the companion, and frequently the intimate friend, of his patient; he must often share his confidence, and, on some occasions, become the depositary of his secrets. His principles, therefore, his knowledge, and his example, become extensively useful or prejudicial. Is he learned, and wise, and good?—his learning will instruct, his skill and his humanity will bless, and his advice and example may amend many among those with whom he daily converses. Is he ignorant, and loose, and debauched? —what mischief may he not do to the younger members of those families who place their confidence in him, and who generally look up to him as a character of superior talent, learning, and worth. Again; the medical character is not only very influential—it is also the most numerous, among the learned professions: the example, therefore, of a physician's knowledge and virtues, or the contamination of his ignorance and his vices, will assume a wider and more extended range.

Is it possible, then, that greater inducements can be offered to a young man, to stimulate his most strenuous exertions, and to call forth all the force of his understanding, and every generous feeling of his heart, than are to be found in the nature, the extent, and the influence of our profession. Occupied on the most important subjects, the ease, the comfort, the happiness, and the lives, of our fellow creatures, it imperiously calls for knowledge and ability. Extensive, beyond the limits of any other science, in the variety of its objects, the continually changing nature of its subjects, and the endless progressive march of its improvements, it is impossible either to acquire what is now known, or to keep pace with its daily accessions of knowledge, but by a zeal and industry as steady and persevering as time itself. Extended over the face of the whole earth, and at the same time penetrating into the recesses of every private family, unless our knowledge be accompanied by prudence, virtue, and religion, we may do more harm by our example, than we can do good by our skill.

Let me then hope, that every young man who now hears me, will lay these important truths seriously to heart; that he will study his profession, not only from motives of ambition and interest, but with a view to the better fulfilment of his moral and religious duties. That he will conscientiously consider the reponsibility of his station, and the influence of his example, and that, whilst he faithfully and respectably fulfils his duty to his patients, by his talents, learning, and industry, he will support the dignity of his own character, by the correctness of his conduct, and recommend his example, by the purity of his manners:—And may peace, reputation, and fortune, be his well-earned reward.

Bei Fragen zur Produktsicherheit wenden Sie sich bitte an:
If you have any questions regarding product safety,
please contact:

Walter de Gruyter GmbH
Genthiner Straße 13
10785 Berlin
productsafety@degruyterbrill.com